Standards Of Emergency Nursing Practice

Fourth Edition

Acknowledgments

Fourth Edition

LEAD EDITOR

Marylou Killian,
RN-c, CS, MS, FNP, CEN
Nurse Practitioner: Emergency Department
The Kingston Hospital
Kingston, NY

EDITORS

T. Randall Huey, RN, MS, CEN
Clinical Nurse Specialist
Piedmont Hospital
Atlanta, GA

Christine Martin, RNA, BSN
Manager, Emergency Services
University of Washington/
Harborview Medical Center
Seattle, WA

Sheila Sanning Shea,
RN, MSN, ANP, CEN
Nurse Practitioner: Emergency Department
Saint Mary Medical Center
Long Beach, CA

ENA STAFF LIAISONS

Nancy Stonis, RN, BSN, MJ, CEN
Director: Professional Services

Tammy Washington
Coordinator: Professional Services

Janice Brown
Coordinator: Professional Services

Sarah Van Sickle
Publication Specialist

Sharon Tarnoff
Group Director: Association Resource
Development and Promotion

Emergency Nurses Association's Mission and Value Statements

The ENA's mission is to provide visionary leadership for emergency nursing and emergency care.

The ENA's mission encompasses the following values:

1. All individuals have a right to quality emergency care delivered with compassion.

2. Respect for diversity of patients and colleagues is inherent to emergency nursing practice and emergency care.

3. Prevention of illness and injury and promotion of wellness are essential components of emergency nursing practice and emergency care.

4. The discipline of emergency nursing includes a defined and evolving body of knowledge based on research.

5. Continuing education and professional development are fundamental to emergency nursing practice and emergency care.

6. Emergency nursing practice is both independent and collaborative.

Emergency Nurses Association's Vision Statement

Defining the Future of Emergency Nursing and Emergency Care through advocacy, expertise, innovation, and leadership.

Contents

Preface

The fourth edition of the Emergency Nurses Association's (ENA's) *Standards of Emergency Nursing Practice (Standards)* was revised in 1998 as part of the cyclical revision of all Emergency Nurses Association documents.

Agencies or individuals who consult this document should understand that these standards represent the philosophy, mission, values, and vision of the Emergency Nurses Association. The standards presented constitute recommended goals and general guidelines of care, education, and experience levels for emergency nurses. The standards do not constitute a legal or regulatory document.

Readers are directed to utilize this Preface and the Introduction to enhance the understanding of specific terms used in the *Standards,* including the "competent" and "excellent" levels.

It should be noted that the term *emergency nurse,* throughout the document, designates a registered professional nurse licensed to practice nursing.

Introduction

HISTORY OF ENA STANDARDS DEVELOPMENT

The ENA's original standards were developed in 1983. The concepts of professionalism, research, education, and practice provided the cornerstone for the development of those standards. The original authors, in concert with ENA leadership, transformed their vision for emergency nursing practice into the philosophy and standards that guide the development of the profession.

The first revision process, completed in 1990, expanded and further defined the original framework and clarified the distinction between competence and excellence, focusing on measurable professional behaviors of the emergency nurse.

The ENA endorsed the 1991 American Nurses Association's (ANA's) *Standards of Clinical Nursing Practice* as generic nursing standards. The third edition of the ENA's *Standards* was completed in 1994. At that time, the ANA's generic standards were adapted as the basis for the further development of emergency nursing specialty standards. The ENA added a triage standard to the standards, because triage is specific to emergency nursing.

RECENT CHANGES IN THE HEALTH CARE ENVIRONMENT THAT AFFECT STANDARDS DEVELOPMENT

The nursing profession is integral to the continuing examination and development of a more cost-effective and efficient health care system. One aspect of nursing's contribution to health care reform is the standards by which the quality of practice, service, and education can be measured.

At present, the health care system is being closely scrutinized. Previously accepted patterns of health care utilization, reimbursement, and treatment are being reexamined. Many organizations and government agencies are involved in the initiative to improve the effectiveness and efficiency of health care. Among these are the American Nurses Association (ANA), the Agency for Health Care Policy and Research (AHCPR), the Joint Commission on the Accreditation of Healthcare Organizations (JCAHO), private insurers, various health care organizations, and other private and government agencies.

The AHCPR is responsible for developing guidelines that will direct clinical practice by providing links among diagnosis, treatments, and outcomes and by describing the alternatives available for each patient. These guidelines, developed by multidisciplinary teams, will serve as frameworks for decision trees that will enable both consumers and providers to make informed treatment choices.

The JCAHO requires hospitals to set standards of patient care with measurable clinical outcomes. The JCAHO defines patient care standards as nursing or medical diagnoses that are directed toward achieving specific patient outcomes.

Professional nursing organizations have developed guidelines and standards that address the nursing care of patients. One of the issues in the development of standards is the lack of consistent terminology. The terms *standards of care, standards of practice,* and *guidelines* have different meanings for different groups. The issue is further complicated by variability in focus and practical application. In this revision, the ENA has addressed the issue of inconsistent terminology by adapting the format used in the ANA's *Standards of Clinical Nursing Practice.*

PRESENTATION OF THE 1998 STANDARDS
The ENA endorsed the 1998 ANA's *Standards of Clinical Nursing Practice 2nd edition* as generic nursing standards. These standards apply to care that is provided to all patients by registered nurses engaged in clinical practice, regardless of clinical specialty, practice setting, or educational preparation (ANA, 1998). These standards of practice are the basis of nursing practice and cannot be subsumed or delegated to individuals not licensed to practice professional nursing. The ANA's *Standards of Clinical Nursing Practice 2nd edition* includes standards of care and standards of professional performance.

AMERICAN NURSES ASSOCIATION STANDARDS OF CLINICAL PRACTICE

Standards of Care

- Assessment
- Diagnosis
- Outcome Identification
- Planning
- Implementation
- Evaluation

Standards of Professional Performance

- Quality of Care
- Performance Appraisal
- Education
- Collegiality
- Ethics
- Collaboration
- Research
- Resource Utilization

In the fourth edition of the Emergency Nurses Association's *Standards,* current American Nurses Association standards are utilized as the foundation for the development of emergency nursing specialty standards. Each comprehensive standard section has been changed to incorporate the term *ANA* for the generic measurement criteria and *ENA* for the specialty measurement criteria. This has been done to facilitate the unification of nursing standards and requisite nomenclature.

A *standard* is an acknowledged measure of quantitative or qualitative value and is designed to set forth a combination of skills, education, and performance that a nurse should strive to achieve. The ANA's standards apply to all nurses in all settings, whereas the specialty standards apply to all nurses practicing in an emergency care setting. The standards are not designed as a legal model to dictate whether an emergency nurse is a competent or an excellent clinician.

The competent level in each standard identifies the levels of performance the emergency nurse, or an institution, should consider in establishing goals for the nurse's professional practice. Each area set forth in the standards does not necessarily have to be met for the nurse's performance to be competent. Competent emergency nursing is demonstrated by sound clinical judgment in autonomous practice.

Emergency nursing at the excellent level is practice that surpasses the competent level and contributes to the growth of emergency nursing practice. Excellent nursing practice may be demonstrated by expert clinical nurses or, in many instances, advanced practice registered nurses (APRNs). The APRN is defined by the ENA as a nurse who has completed a master's degree in a specialty area of nursing and is clinically active in that specialty. The excellence standards have been amended to better demonstrate the contributions of APRNs in the emergency setting and their role in increasingly complex patient care.

It is important to remember, in the evaluation of competence or excellence, that total performance should be evaluated over time and in relation to specific events and individual environments. The ENA has taken the position that entry level into nursing practice should be at the baccalaureate level. The ENA also believes that participation in the professional organization is a key factor in the development of professional nurses.

The ENA recognizes that different terms are being used in the health care environment to refer to the people served (e.g., *patient, client, consumer,* and *customer*). The ENA has chosen to refer those served by emergency nurses as *patients.* The *Standards of Emergency Nursing Practice* have been developed in accordance with the ENA's mission and value statements concerning respect for diversity of patients and colleagues as an inherent and integral part of professional practice. The ENA's Standards of Care are therefore applicable to all patients and reflect the varied population encountered in emergency settings. A patient's age, race, gender, culture, or sexual orientation does not preclude the use of these *Standards* in the development of a plan of care. The ENA's Standards of Professional Performance apply to all clinicians, including clinical nurses, nurse educators, advanced practice nurses, and nurses practicing in a management role.

The following is the format for this revision of the *Standards of Emergency Nursing Practice* fourth edition:

• Statement of the ANA's generic standard.

• Statement of the specialty standard.

• Rationale for the specialty standard.

• Statement of the ANA's generic standard measurement criteria.

• Statement of the ENA's measurement criteria at the competent and excellent levels.

Criteria including key indicators of competent and excellent practice have been, and will continue to be, revised on a cyclical basis to incorporate advances in scientific knowledge, clinical practice, and technology.

SUMMARY

Since 1983, the *Standards of Emergency Nursing Practice* has been a springboard for growth within a dynamic emergency nursing environment. As such, it continues to be used for a variety of purposes:

- Development of criteria-based job descriptions

- Guidance of criteria-based performance evaluations

- Development of departmental policies and procedures

- Development of standardized emergency care plans

- Guidance of interviewing and hiring practices for emergency nurses

- Development of orientation, in-service, and continuing education programs

- Creation and revision of emergency care forms

- Development of quality improvement programs and activities

- Development of curricula for baccalaureate and graduate emergency nursing programs

- Support of reimbursement for nursing care

- Integration of standards and guidelines into the blueprint for the Certification Examination for Emergency Nurses

- As a resource document for a variety of other ENA publications

Emergency Nurses Association Standards of Care

The following section delineates the ENA's Standards of Care which include:

The format of each subsection includes generic standards and specialty standards. The generic standards are published by the ANA in *Standards of Clinical Practice, 2nd edition* (1998) and are applicable to all nurses.

The specialty standards and measurement criteria are derivations of the generic standards and criteria. They specifically define how an emergency nurse should perform at the competent and excellent levels.

Comprehensive Standard I
Assessment

ANA Standard*
The nurse collects patient health data.

Specialty Standard
The emergency nurse initiates accurate and ongoing assessment of physical and psychosocial concerns of patients within the emergency care system.

Rationale
Assessment is a series of systematic, organized, and deliberate actions to identify and obtain data about the patient. This assessment provides the database for determination of the state of health or illness of the patient.

AMERICAN NURSES ASSOCIATION MEASUREMENT CRITERIA*

1. Data collection involves the patient, family, and other health care providers as appropriate.

2. The priority of data collection activities is determined by the patient's immediate condition or needs.

3. Pertinent data are collected using appropriate assessment techniques and instruments.

4. Relevant data are documented in a retrievable form.

5. The data collection process is systematic and ongoing.

* Reprinted with permission from American Nurses Association, *Standards of Clinical Nursing Practice,*
2nd edition. ©1998 American Nurses Publishing, American Nurses Foundation/American Nurses Association,
600 Maryland Avenue, SW, Suite 100 West, Washington, DC 20024-2571.

EMERGENCY NURSES ASSOCIATION MEASUREMENT CRITERIA

A systematic and pertinent collection of data about the health status of every patient is assessed.

Competent Level

- Obtains initial focused subjective and objective data through history taking, physical examination, review of records, and communication with health care providers and families, as appropriate.

- Conducts assessment within the framework of holistic professional nursing practice.

- Performs the initial assessment based on the patient's presentation. Ongoing assessments are performed as established by departmental policies and as warranted by the patient's response.

- Uses assessment techniques and criteria that are pertinent to the patient's age-specific physical, developmental, cognitive, and psychosocial needs.

- Records relevant data for every patient in a retrievable form, as appropriate to the nature and severity of illness or injury.

- Communicates significant data to appropriate personnel throughout the patient's emergency care experience.

- Assesses the patient's and the family's learning needs.

Excellent Level

- Obtains initial and thorough subjective and objective data through history taking, physical examination, review of records, and communication with health care providers, significant others, and caretakers as appropriate.

- Serves as a role model and resource person to facilitate the performance of accurate and ongoing nursing assessments.

- Identifies nursing or system deficiencies that may impede adequate assessment.

- Is identified as a resource for consultation among peers and/or other health care colleagues in the community.

Comprehensive Standard II
Diagnosis

ANA Standard*
The nurse analyzes assessment data in determining diagnoses.

Specialty Standard
The emergency nurse analyzes assessment data to formulate nursing diagnoses and identify collaborative problems for each patient and/or family.

Rationale
Use of diagnostic reasoning in the analysis of assessment data helps determine the patient's health status.

AMERICAN NURSES ASSOCIATION MEASUREMENT CRITERIA*

1. Diagnoses are derived from the assessment data.

2. Diagnoses are validated with the patient, families, and other health care providers, when possible and appropriate.

3. Diagnoses are documented in a manner that facilitates the determination of expected outcomes and plan of care.

* Reprinted with permission from American Nurses Association, *Standards of Clinical Nursing Practice, 2nd edition.* ©1998 American Nurses Publishing, American Nurses Foundation/American Nurses Association, 600 Maryland Avenue, SW, Suite 100 West, Washington, DC 20024-2571.

EMERGENCY NURSES ASSOCIATION MEASUREMENT CRITERIA

For every patient, the emergency nurse identifies the actual and potential problems or nursing diagnoses based on pertinent data collected in the focused assessment.

Competent Level

- Identifies nursing diagnoses and/or collaborative problems, based on defining characteristics, that is, signs and symptoms recognized during a focused, systematic assessment.

- Utilizes assessment data from pertinent sources to identify collaborative problems and formulate nursing diagnoses.

- Communicates and validates nursing diagnoses with other health care providers, as appropriate.

- Identifies and communicates collaborative problems to other health care providers, as appropriate.

- Documents nursing diagnoses and/or collaborative problems in a retrievable form.

- Identifies actual or potential knowledge deficits for the patient and the family.

Excellent Level

- Anticipates and recognizes nursing diagnoses, collaborative problems, and/or medical diagnosis based on atypical or subtle defining characteristics as appropriate for the nurse's legal scope of practice.

- Identifies challenges that may impede adequate identification of nursing diagnoses and/or collaborative problems.

- Participates in the development and implementation of tools and systems to facilitate effective use of nursing diagnoses.

- Clinically tests nursing diagnoses in emergency nursing for appropriateness and relevance.

- Validates nursing and/or medical diagnoses for specific emergency patients and patient populations as defined by the nurse's legal scope of practice.

Comprehensive Standard III
Outcome Identification

ANA Standard*
The nurse identifies expected outcomes individualized to the patient.

Specialty Standard
The emergency nurse identifies expected outcomes individualized to the emergency patient based on assessment, nursing diagnoses, collaborative problems, and/or medical diagnosis.

Rationale
Outcome identification is the bridge from assessment and nursing diagnoses to intervention and evaluation, providing focus and clarity to the plan of care.

AMERICAN NURSES ASSOCIATION MEASUREMENT CRITERIA*

1. Outcomes are derived from the diagnoses.

2. Outcomes are mutually formulated with the patient, family, and other health care providers, when possible and appropriate.

3. Outcomes are culturally appropriate and realistic in relation to the patient's present and potential capabilities.

4. Outcomes are attainable in relation to resources available to the patient.

5. Outcomes include a time estimate for attainment.

6. Outcomes provide direction for continuity of care.

7. Outcomes are documented as measurable goals.

* Reprinted with permission from American Nurses Association, *Standards of Clinical Nursing Practice*, *2nd edition.* ©1998 American Nurses Publishing, American Nurses Foundation/American Nurses Association, 600 Maryland Avenue, SW, Suite 100 West, Washington, DC 20024-2571.

EMERGENCY NURSES ASSOCIATION MEASUREMENT CRITERIA

Physical and psychosocial outcomes are identified for each patient as appropriate.

Competent Level

- Identifies measurable short-term and long-term outcomes.

- Identifies appropriate time frames for attainment of outcomes related to the patient's nursing diagnoses and/or collaborative problems.

- Communicates expected outcomes to other health care providers, the patient, and the family to ensure continuity of care.

- Utilizes Nursing Outcomes Classification (NOC) to communicate expected outcomes to other health care providers to ensure continuity of care, when appropriate.

Excellent Level

- Acts as a resource for the development of an outcome-driven plan of care for each patient.

- Develops peer education that emphasizes identification and utilization of patient outcome measures.

- Develops clinical guidelines and/or critical pathways of expected outcomes for groups of patients with similar diagnoses and /or collaborative problems and shares this expertise with other health care providers.

Comprehensive Standard IV
Planning

ANA Standard*
The nurse develops a plan of care that prescribes interventions to attain expected outcomes.

Specialty Standard
The emergency nurse formulates a plan of care with the emergency patient and/or family based on: assessment; nursing diagnoses; collaborative problems; identified outcomes; and/or medical diagnosis, within the nurse's legal scope of practice.

Rationale
Safe, effective, and fiscally responsible emergency patient care results from active, focused planning by the emergency nurse.

AMERICAN NURSES ASSOCIATION MEASUREMENT CRITERIA*

1. The plan is individualized to the patient (e.g., age-appropriate, culturally sensitive) and the patient's condition or needs.

2. The plan is developed with the patient, family, and other health care providers, as appropriate.

3. The plan reflects current nursing practice.

4. The plan provides for continuity of care.

5. Priorities for care are established.

6. The plan is documented.

* Reprinted with permission from American Nurses Association, *Standards of Clinical Nursing Practice, 2nd edition.* ©1998 American Nurses Publishing, American Nurses Foundation/American Nurses Association, 600 Maryland Avenue, SW, Suite 100 West, Washington, DC 20024-2571.

EMERGENCY NURSES ASSOCIATION MEASUREMENT CRITERIA

The plan of care for the emergency patient is systematic and consistent with safe, effective, and fiscally responsible patient care.

Competent Level

- Develops a plan of care for each patient based on current scientific knowledge, recognizing diversity, that addresses nursing diagnosis and/or collaborative problems.

- Collaborates with the patient, the family, and appropriate heath care providers in developing the plan of care.

- Identifies priorities for nursing actions, patient goals, and patient outcomes.

- Prescribes interventions as appropriate for the nurse's legal scope of practice.

- Addresses environmental, physical, developmental, and psychosocial stressors in the plan of care.

- Incorporates teaching and learning principles in the plan of care, based on identified learning needs and developmental level.

- Communicates the plan of care to other health care providers, the patient, and the patient's family to ensure continuity of care.

- Utilizes Nursing Interventions Classification (NIC) to communicate the plan of care, as appropriate.

- Ensures that the plan of care is family centered.

Excellent Level

- Develops, implements, and evaluates materials for patient care and education.

- Acts as a resource for the use of patient care guidelines and/or critical pathways.

- Participates in the development, implementation, and evaluation of tools to facilitate care planning, such as guidelines or clinical and/or critical pathways.

- Designs the departmental framework to facilitate involvement of the patient and significant others in the plan of care.

- Develops a plan of care that addresses potential nursing diagnoses and/or collaborative problems based on changing patient status.

- Develops a plan of care that recognizes the implications of the patient's long-term problems.

Comprehensive Standard V
Implementation

ANA Standard*
The nurse implements the interventions identified in the plan of care.

Specialty Standard
The emergency nurse implements a plan of care based on assessment, nursing diagnoses and/or collaborative problems, and outcome identification.

Rationale
Assessment data, nursing diagnoses and/or collaborative problems, outcome criteria, and planning provide a foundation for implementation of interventions.

AMERICAN NURSES ASSOCIATION MEASUREMENT CRITERIA*

1. Interventions are consistent with the established plan of care.

2. Interventions are implemented in a safe, timely, and appropriate manner.

3. Interventions are documented.

* Reprinted with permission from American Nurses Association, *Standards of Clinical Nursing Practice, 2nd edition.* ©1998 American Nurses Publishing, American Nurses Foundation/American Nurses Association, 600 Maryland Avenue, SW, Suite 100 West, Washington, DC 20024-2571.

EMERGENCY NURSES ASSOCIATION MEASUREMENT CRITERIA

Interventions are prioritized based on the patient's needs and consideration of the patient's family.

Competent Level

- Implements the plan of care for each patient.

- Performs appropriate patient monitoring.

- Provides education to the patient and the family regarding current health status or condition and discharge teaching, as appropriate.

- Anticipates the need for additional resources to implement interventions.

- Works collaboratively with other health care providers, as appropriate, to implement interventions.

- Utilizes Nursing Interventions Classification (NIC) to document performed interventions, as appropriate.

Excellent Level

- Identifies and independently performs appropriate interventions.

- Works collaboratively with other health care providers, as appropriate, to implement more complex interventions.

Comprehensive Standard VI
Evaluation

ANA Standard*
The nurse evaluates the patient's progress toward attainment of outcomes.

Specialty Standard
The emergency nurse evaluates and modifies the plan of care based on observable patient responses and attainment of expected outcomes.

Rationale
The dynamic nature of emergency patient care requires continual evaluation to optimize achievement of patient outcomes.

AMERICAN NURSES ASSOCIATION MEASUREMENT CRITERIA*

1. Evaluation is systematic, ongoing, and criterion-based.

2. The patient, family, and other health care providers are involved in the evaluation process, as appropriate.

3. Ongoing assessment data are used to revise diagnoses, outcomes, and the plan of care as needed.

4. Revisions in diagnoses, outcomes, and the plan of care are documented.

5. The effectiveness of interventions is evaluated in relation to outcomes.

6. The patient's responses to interventions are documented.

* Reprinted with permission from American Nurses Association, *Standards of Clinical Nursing Practice,*
2nd edition. ©1998 American Nurses Publishing, American Nurses Foundation/American Nurses Association,
600 Maryland Avenue, SW, Suite 100 West, Washington, DC 20024-2571.

EMERGENCY NURSES ASSOCIATION MEASUREMENT CRITERIA

The patient's response to interventions is continually evaluated to determine progress toward resolution of immediate needs.

Competent Level

- Utilizes current patient data to measure progress toward attainment of patient outcomes.

- Utilizes data from the patient, significant others, and other health care providers to evaluate the patient's responses to intervention.

- Documents the patient's response to interventions and changes in the patient's condition and modifies the plan of care as appropriate.

- Evaluates progress toward achievement of expected outcomes, modifying interventions and/or outcomes as appropriate.

- Modifies outcomes, as needed, through discussion with the patient and the family when changes occur in the patient's status and available resources.

- Communicates evaluation to other health care team members, as appropriate, to achieve desired outcomes.

Excellent Level

- Performs comprehensive evaluation of the patient's care and education.

- Functions as a resource person for evaluation of patient care.

Comprehensive Standard VII
Triage

ANA Standard
None

Specialty Standard
The emergency nurse triages each patient and determines the priority of care based on physical, developmental, and psychosocial needs, as well as factors influencing access to health care and patient flow through the emergency care system.*

Rationale
Triage facilitates the flow of patients through the emergency care system to ensure timely evaluation of patient needs.

---

*The ENA believes that safe, effective, and efficient triage can be performed only by a registered professional nurse who is educated in the principles of triage and who has a minimum of 6 months' experience in emergency nursing.

EMERGENCY NURSES ASSOCIATION MEASUREMENT CRITERIA

1. Assessment: A rapid, systematic collection of data relevant to each patient's chief complaint, age, cognitive level, and social situation is conducted to obtain sufficient information to determine patient acuity and any immediate physical or psychosocial needs.

Competent Level

- Performs focused assessment of chief complaint on each patient entering the emergency care system, collecting subjective and objective data.

- Assesses patients in a timely manner according to established triage criteria.

- Documents the triage assessment, including appropriate subjective and objective data.

Excellent Level

- Serves as a role model and resource person in the assessment phase of triage.

- Participates in development, implementation, and/or revision of triage assessment systems, such as age-specific guidelines and complaint-specific protocols.

- Participates in development, implementation, and/or revision of tools for documenting the triage assessment.

2. Diagnosis: *Information gathered in the assessment phase is analyzed to determine the severity of physical, psychosocial, and educational needs.*

Competent Level

- Differentiates the severity of the patient's condition.

- Identifies nursing diagnoses and/or collaborative problems when possible.

- Documents clinical impressions.

Excellent Level

- Recognizes nursing diagnoses and/or collaborative problems using atypical or subtle defining characteristics.

- Acts as role model and resource person for triage confirmation, identification of collaborative problems, and/or validation of nursing diagnoses.

3. Outcome Identification: *Individualized expected outcomes are identified for each patient.*

Competent Level

- Formulates outcomes relative to nursing diagnoses and/or collaborative problems, available resources, the patient's abilities, and input from the patient and other health care providers.

- Identifies and documents measurable objective criteria.

Excellent Level

- Addresses atypical presentations to identify patients at high risk for adverse outcomes.

- Acts as a role model and resource person for confirmation and validation of outcome identification.

4. Planning: *The urgency of physical, psychosocial, and educational needs is determined, and the course of action is formulated to attain expected outcomes.*

Competent Level

- Differentiates the urgency of the patient's problems and prioritizes access to care based on the patient's acuity.

- Directs the patient to the appropriate treatment area, based on assessment, diagnoses, outcome identification, and acuity.

- Communicates pertinent information to other health care providers.

- Documents the acuity and the individual plan of care.

- Identifies interventions to attain expected outcomes.

Excellent Level

- Anticipates the patient's needs and interventions, based on identification of actual and high-risk health problems.

- Acts as a role model and resource person for the planning phase of triage.

5. *Implementation:* **Interventions are implemented as identified in the plan of care.

Competent Level

- Initiates independent nursing measures.
- Initiates diagnostic procedures per established triage protocols.
- Initiates treatment per established protocols, for example, antipyretics.
- Documents all interventions.
- Communicates pertinent information to the patient and significant others.
- Mobilizes additional resources as needed.

Excellent Level

- Participates in development and implementation of independent nursing measures and collaborative protocols.
- Identifies implementation practices requiring modification or change.
- Acts as a role model and a resource person for independent and collaborative interventions.

6. Evaluation: *The patient's response to intervention is evaluated.*

Competent Level

- Reassesses the patient according to the acuity and established procedures.

- Evaluates and documents the effectiveness of all interventions, as appropriate.

- Modifies the plan of care, acuity, and the expected outcome based on new information or changes in assessment data.

Excellent Level

- Acts as a role model and resource person for the evaluation phase of the triage process.

- Identifies nursing or system deficiencies that may impede adequate evaluation of the patient.

7. Medical Screening Examinations: *The emergency nurse offers medical screening examinations as defined by institutional policies and state and federal regulations.*

Competent Level

- Promotes access to care through appropriate screening of patients in accordance with the Emergency Medical Treatment and Active Labor Act (EMTALA) and state regulations.

Excellent Level

- Participates in the development of policies related to screening examinations.

- Coordinates staff education related to medical screening examinations.

Emergency Nurses Association Standards of Professional Performance

The following section delineates the ENA's Standards of Professional Performance which include:

The format of each subsection includes generic standards and specialty standards. The generic standards are published by the ANA in *Standards of Clinical Nursing Practice, 2nd edition* (ANA, 1998), and are applicable to all nurses.

The specialty standards and measurement criteria are derivations of the generic standards and criteria. They specifically define how an emergency nurse should perform at the competent and excellent levels.

Comprehensive Standard VIII
Quality of Care

ANA Standard*
The nurse systematically evaluates the quality and effectiveness of nursing practice.

Specialty Standard
The emergency nurse evaluates the quality and effectiveness of emergency nursing practice.

Rationale
Evaluation of emergency nursing practice is a continuous process to ensure that quality of care is improved.

AMERICAN NURSES ASSOCIATION MEASUREMENT CRITERIA*

1. The nurse participates in quality of care activities as appropriate to the nurse's education and position. Such activities may include:
   - identification of aspects of care important for quality monitoring
   - analysis of quality data to identify opportunities for improving care
   - development of policies, procedures, and practice guidelines to improve quality of care
   - identification of indicators used to monitor quality and effectiveness of nursing care
   - collection of data to monitor quality and effectiveness of nursing care
   - formulation of recommendations to improve nursing practice or patient outcomes
   - implementation of activities to enhance the quality of nursing practice
   - participation on interdisciplinary teams that evaluate clinical practice or health services

* Reprinted with permission from American Nurses Association, *Standards of Clinical Nursing Practice, 2nd edition.* ©1998 American Nurses Publishing, American Nurses Foundation/American Nurses Association, 600 Maryland Avenue, SW, Suite 100 West, Washington, DC 20024-2571.

2. The nurse uses the results of quality of care activities to initiate changes in nursing practice.

3. The nurse uses the results of quality of care activities to initiate changes throughout the health care delivery system, as appropriate.

EMERGENCY NURSES ASSOCIATION MEASUREMENT CRITERIA

1. The emergency nurse develops and implements a comprehensive plan for assessing and improving the quality of care for emergency patients.

Competent Level

- Participates in the development and implementation of the plan for assessing and improving quality of care for emergency patients.

- Participates in the development and implementation of actions, resolutions, and ongoing monitoring activities designed to improve emergency nursing practice and the health care system.

- Communicates and documents quality of care issues.

Excellent Level

- Works collaboratively to develop, implement, and evaluate a multidisciplinary quality assessment and improvement plan.

- Implements and evaluates actions, resolutions, and ongoing indicators designed to improve emergency nursing practice.

- Develops, implements, and evaluates quality of care actions to monitor indicators for emergency nursing excellence.

- Develops, implements, and evaluates methods to enhance the quality of nursing care.

- Initiates mechanisms to address quality of care issues.

- Monitors regulatory and legislative activities that affect the quality of emergency nursing practice.

- Participates in collaborative quality assessment and improvement activities.

2. The emergency nurse continually assesses and evaluates the care delivery system using quality improvement principles and practices.

Competent Level

- Identifies internal and external customers, including patients, physicians, staff, other departments, and community agencies.

- Assesses customer needs to maximize customer satisfaction.

- Continuously collaborates with other departments to improve and enhance the delivery of patient care.

- Participates in system analysis and redesign to increase efficiency and productivity.

Excellent Level

- Acts as a resource for quality improvement principles and methods.

- Develops customer satisfaction surveys, analyzes results, and makes recommendations for change, as appropriate.

- Participates in and/or leads multidisciplinary quality action teams.

- Develops, implements, and evaluates system analysis plans to increase efficiency and productivity.

Comprehensive Standard IX
Performance Appraisal

ANA Standard*
The nurse evaluates one's own nursing practice in relation to professional practice standards and relevant statutes and regulations.

Specialty Standard
The emergency nurse adheres to established standards of practice, including activities and behaviors that characterize professional status.

Rationale
Safe and effective nursing practice depends on the application of a specific body of knowledge and skills congruent with professional behavior.

AMERICAN NURSES ASSOCIATION MEASUREMENT CRITERIA*

1. The nurse engages in performance appraisal on a regular basis, identifying areas of strength as well as areas where professional development would be beneficial.

2. The nurse seeks constructive feedback regarding one's own practice.

3. The nurse takes action to achieve goals identified during performance appraisal.

4. The nurse participates in peer review as appropriate.

5. The nurse's practice reflects knowledge of current professional practice standards, laws, and regulations.

* Reprinted with permission from American Nurses Association, *Standards of Clinical Nursing Practice, 2nd edition.* ©1998 American Nurses Publishing, American Nurses Foundation/American Nurses Association, 600 Maryland Avenue, SW, Suite 100 West, Washington, DC 20024-2571.

EMERGENCY NURSES ASSOCIATION MEASUREMENT CRITERIA

1. The emergency nurse is accountable for his or her own actions.

Competent Level

- Assumes responsibility for his or her actions.
- Possesses a knowledge base related to:
  - collection and processing of data related to physical, psychosocial, spiritual, and developmental needs of each patient and family.
  - identification of nursing diagnoses.
  - identification of outcomes.
  - development and implementation of a plan of care.
  - evaluation of care based on observable responses.
- Understands regulatory and legislative issues that affect the practice of emergency nursing.

Excellent Level

- Utilizes authority and responsibility to provide competency-based job descriptions and nursing performance reviews.
- Monitors regulatory and legislative activities that affect the practice of the emergency nurse and utilizes those key issues as a part of the performance appraisal process.

2. The emergency nurse participates in clinical and peer review to evaluate practice.

Competent Level

- Uses self-evaluation, peer evaluation, and feedback from health care providers and others to modify and improve practice.

Excellent Level

- Plans, initiates, and evaluates clinical care and the peer review process to assess professional practice.
- Develops, implements, and evaluates programs of competency-based performance appraisal.

Comprehensive Standard X
Education

ANA Standard*
The nurse acquires and maintains current knowledge and competency in nursing practice.

Specialty Standard
The emergency nurse recognizes self-learning needs and opportunities and is accountable for maximizing professional development and optimal emergency nursing practice.

Rationale
Inherent to the process of continuing education is the responsibility for self-learning and integration of that learning into daily practice.

AMERICAN NURSES ASSOCIATION MEASUREMENT CRITERIA*

1. The nurse participates in ongoing educational activities related to clinical knowledge and professional issues.

2. The nurse seeks experiences that reflect current clinical practice in order to maintain current clinical skills and competence.

3. The nurse acquires knowledge and skills appropriate to the specialty area and practice setting.

* Reprinted with permission from American Nurses Association, *Standards of Clinical Nursing Practice,*
2nd edition. ©1998 American Nurses Publishing, American Nurses Foundation/American Nurses Association,
600 Maryland Avenue, SW, Suite 100 West, Washington, DC 20024-2571.

EMERGENCY NURSES ASSOCIATION CRITERIA

1. The emergency nurse is responsible for acquiring and demonstrating attainment of a defined body of emergency nursing knowledge.

Competent Level

- Completes appropriate orientation to the emergency care area.

- Demonstrates knowledge and skills required for stabilization and/or treatment of the emergency patient.

- Attains Basic Life Support provider status.

- Attains Advanced Cardiac Life Support and/or Pediatric Advanced Life Support provider status, as appropriate.

- Attains Certification in Emergency Nursing (CEN®).

- Attains Trauma Nursing Core Course (TNCC) provider status (minimum level of education for emergency nurses caring for trauma patients).

- Attains Emergency Nursing Pediatric Course (ENPC) provider status (minimum level of education for emergency nurses caring for pediatric patients).

- Acts as a clinical preceptor for students and orientees.

Excellent Level

- Serves as a role model for clinical preceptors.

- Acts as a resource person for clinical preceptors.

- Provides continuing education related to the specialty of emergency nursing.

- Contributes relevant information to the literature.

- Attains Advanced Cardiac Life Support and/or Pediatric Advanced Life Support instructor status (recommended).

- Attains TNCC instructor status (recommended).

- Attains ENPC instructor status (recommended).

- Attends Concepts in Advanced Trauma Nursing.

- Develops, implements, monitors, and evaluates competency-based staff education.

- Coordinates and directs preceptor programs.

2. The emergency nurse obtains ongoing education consistent with the role and area of practice.

Competent Level

- Determines professional learning needs and identifies short- and long-term educational goals relevant to his or her own practice.

- Plans and implements activities to achieve educational goals.

- Shares newly gained knowledge from relevant educational programs with peers.

- Applies knowledge and skills learned through continuing education to improve clinical practice.

- Participates in the development and implementation of tools, systems, and techniques that enhance nursing assessment and documentation.

- Participates in community education programs.

- Continues formal education.

Excellent Level

- Exceeds educational activities necessary to meet minimal institutional requirements or requirements for continuing licensure.

- Acts as a role model and a resource person to facilitate and validate the analysis of assessment data for accurate and appropriate identification of nursing diagnoses and/or collaborative problems.

- Recommends practice or system changes based on analysis of current trends.

- Plans and implements community education programs.

Comprehensive Standard XI
Collegiality

ANA Standard*
The nurse interacts with, and contributes to the professional development of, peers and other health care providers as colleagues.

Specialty Standard
The emergency nurse engages in activities and behaviors that characterize a professional.

Rationale
To promote nursing as a profession and emergency nursing as a specialty, the emergency nurse identifies and demonstrates behaviors congruent with professional status.

AMERICAN NURSES ASSOCIATION MEASUREMENT CRITERIA*

1. The nurse shares knowledge and skills with colleagues.

2. The nurse provides peers with constructive feedback regarding their practice.

3. The nurse interacts with colleagues to enhance one's own professional nursing practice.

4. The nurse contributes to an environment that is conducive to the clinical education of nursing students, other health care students, and other employees, as appropriate.

5. The nurse contributes to a supportive and healthy work environment.

* Reprinted with permission from American Nurses Association, *Standards of Clinical Nursing Practice*, *2nd edition.* ©1998 American Nurses Publishing, American Nurses Foundation/American Nurses Association, 600 Maryland Avenue, SW, Suite 100 West, Washington, DC 20024-2571.

EMERGENCY NURSES ASSOCIATION MEASUREMENT CRITERIA

1. The emergency nurse supports the professional development of nursing by promoting understanding of nursing roles and responsibilities.

Competent Level

- Identifies self and role to patients and significant others.

- Identifies self to colleagues and other health care providers.

- Utilizes collegial relationships to influence patient outcomes and care delivery within the health care system.

- Becomes a participating member of the ENA.

- Participates as a professional nurse in community activities.

Excellent Level

- Assumes leadership roles in the ENA.

- Serves as a liaison for internal and external groups, such as professional organizations, academic and health care institutions, and community health care agencies.

2. The emergency nurse possesses an understanding of current and proposed legislation and regulations related to emergency care and the practice of emergency nursing.

Competent Level

- Pursues knowledge of current and proposed regulations and legislation relating to health care issues.

- Utilizes knowledge of legislation and regulations to plan patient care.

- Adheres to legislation and regulations related to emergency care.

- Pursues knowledge regarding the ENA's position on health care policies.

Excellent Level

- Participates in activities to promote internal regulation of the profession and autonomous practice.

- Monitors and participates in legislative activities that affect emergency nursing practice and health care issues.

3. The emergency nurse fosters a professional image of nursing.

Competent Level

- Demonstrates a professional image to patients, significant others, peers, other health care providers, the media, and the public.

- Acts as a mentor for potential nurses to encourage entry into nursing.

Excellent Level

- Functions within a leadership role to articulate and demonstrate the professional role of the emergency nurse to patients, significant others, peers, other health care providers, the media, and the public.

- Acts as a mentor to nursing peers to encourage professional growth.

4. The emergency nurse has responsibility for public education regarding emergency nursing and the emergency care system.

Competent Level

- Disseminates information regarding emergency nursing.

Excellent Level

- Plans and/or participates in community activities to educate consumers about emergency nursing and emergency care.

- Communicates with legislators regarding public policy as it relates to public education and awareness of emergency nursing and emergency care issues.

5. The emergency nurse facilitates learning experiences for peers, other health care providers, students, and volunteers.

Competent Level

- Acts as a teacher, role model, preceptor, and mentor.

- Facilitates the learning of professional nursing students regarding the roles and responsibilities of emergency nurses.

- Educates peers and other health care providers about the roles and responsibilities of the emergency nurse.

- Participates in the orientation of students, peers, volunteers, and other health care providers.

- Participates in the education and supervision of students and other health care providers during clinical practice, as appropriate.

Excellent Level

- Develops, implements, and evaluates orientation programs, preceptorship, mentoring programs, and education programs related to emergency nursing.

- Participates in the planning, implementation, and evaluation of multidisciplinary educational activities.

6. *The emergency nurse promotes wellness in the workplace.*

Competent Level

- Participates in wellness programs within institutions.
- Identifies personal stressors or illness and modifies behaviors in response to identified personal concerns.

Excellent Level

- Formulates departmental or institutional plans to promote wellness programs.
- Assists personnel in identifying personal stressors and refers them to appropriate resources.

Comprehensive Standard XII
Ethics

ANA Standard*
The nurse's decisions and actions on behalf of patients are determined in an ethical manner.

Specialty Standard
The emergency nurse provides care based on philosophical and ethical concepts. These concepts include reverence for life; respect for the inherent dignity, worth, autonomy, and individuality of each human being; and an acknowledgment of the diversity of all people.

Rationale
The belief in human worth makes up the philosophical foundation on which nursing is based.

AMERICAN NURSES ASSOCIATION MEASUREMENT CRITERIA*

1. The nurse's practice is guided by the *Code for Nurses*.

2. The nurse maintains patient confidentiality within legal and regulatory parameters.

3. The nurse acts as a patient advocate and assists patients in developing skills so they can advocate for themselves.

4. The nurse delivers care in a nonjudgmental and nondiscriminatory manner that is sensitive to patient diversity.

5. The nurse delivers care in a manner that preserves patient autonomy, dignity, and rights.

6. The nurse seeks available resources in formulating ethical decisions.

* Reprinted with permission from American Nurses Association, *Standards of Clinical Nursing Practice, 2nd edition.* ©1998 American Nurses Publishing, American Nurses Foundation/American Nurses Association, 600 Maryland Avenue, SW, Suite 100 West, Washington, DC 20024-2571.

EMERGENCY NURSES ASSOCIATION MEASUREMENT CRITERIA

1. The emergency nurse provides care that demonstrates ethical beliefs and respect for patients' rights.

Competent Level

- Respects the individuality and human worth of patients, regardless of age, gender, sexual orientation, socioeconomic status, cultural or ethnic background, spiritual and ethical beliefs, marginalization, or the nature of health problems.

- Respects the dignity, confidentiality, and privacy of patients.

- Serves as an advocate for the patient and significant others.

Excellent Level

- Participates on the institution's and departmental ethics committees.

- Participates in the development and implementation of policies and procedures as they relate to ethical issues in emergency care.

- Develops, implements, and evaluates programs related to ethical issues in emergency care.

- Participates in the development and implementation of education to increase community awareness of advanced directives legislation.

- Acts as a role model for ethical practice.

2. The emergency nurse functions autonomously to the extent that knowledge, skills, and role permit.

Competent Level

- Acts congruently with institutional and professional practice standards and state nursing practice acts.

Excellent Level

- Initiates case and peer review to evaluate autonomous practice.

3. The emergency nurse exercises authority congruent with the state nursing practice act and is knowledgeable of local, state, and federal laws that govern the delivery of care.

Competent Level

- Complies with the state nursing practice act, policies and procedures of the institution, and local, state, and federal statutes.

- Coordinates delivery of patient care.

- Informs the patient of legal rights, as required.

- Ensures that informed consent is obtained for each patient, as appropriate.

- Follows appropriate policies and procedures when a patient is physically restrained or treated on an involuntary basis.

- Advocates for the patient's rights as delineated by advanced directives, durable powers-of-attorney, and other documents that address end-of-life issues.

- Understands and complies with interfacility transfer guidelines, as mandated by the Consolidated Omnibus Budget Reconciliation Act of 1986 (COBRA)/Emergency Medical Treatment and Active Labor Act (EMTALA) legislation.

- Utilizes authority and responsibility as the ultimate decision-maker on issues regarding emergency nursing, maintaining accountability for this decision making.

Excellent Level

- Assumes leadership roles in clinical and managerial situations.

- Defines standards of emergency nursing practice within the institution and area of practice.

- Participates in the development and education of policies and procedures related to the legal responsibilities of the emergency nurse.

Comprehensive Standard XIII
Collaboration

ANA Standard*
The nurse collaborates with the patient, family, and other health care providers in providing patient care.

Specialty Standard
The emergency nurse ensures open and timely communication with emergency patients, significant others, and other health care providers through professional collaboration.

Rationale
Effective communication with the patient, significant others, and other health care providers promotes positive health practices within the institution and the community.

AMERICAN NURSES ASSOCIATION MEASUREMENT CRITERIA*

1. The nurse communicates with the patient, family, and other health care providers regarding patient care and nursing's role in the provision of care.

2. The nurse collaborates with the patient, family, and other health care providers in the formulation of overall goals and the plan of care, and in decisions related to care and the delivery of services.

3. The nurse consults with other health care providers for patient care, as needed.

4. The nurse makes referrals, including provisions for continuity of care, as needed.

* Reprinted with permission from American Nurses Association, *Standards of Clinical Nursing Practice, 2nd edition.* ©1998 American Nurses Publishing, American Nurses Foundation/American Nurses Association, 600 Maryland Avenue, SW, Suite 100 West, Washington, DC 20024-2571.

EMERGENCY NURSES ASSOCIATION MEASUREMENT CRITERIA

1. The emergency nurse ensures open communication with the patient and significant others.

Competent Level

- Provides pertinent information to the patient and significant others to enhance the decision-making process.

Excellent Level

- Acts as a resource and a role model to promote involvement of the patient and significant others in the decision-making process.

2. The emergency nurse participates in community education related to emergency care.

Competent Level

- Participates in community education related to emergency nursing and emergency care systems.
- Participates in community education related to injury and illness prevention.

Excellent Level

- Plans, implements, and evaluates appropriate educational offerings at the community level.
- Utilizes patient outcome data to develop prevention and/or education programs.

3. The emergency nurse utilizes education of the patient and significant others to clarify learning needs and optimize patient outcomes.

Competent Level

- Provides information about the patient's condition to the patient and significant others, as appropriate, in a way that is consistent with their intellectual, developmental, and emotional abilities.

- Provides explanations about treatments before their initiation, whenever possible.

- Involves patients and significant others in the decision-making process related to therapeutic interventions, whenever possible.

- Explains or ensures explanation of medications, treatments, self-care, referral, and/or prevention.

- Provides and explains written instructions regarding after care, follow-up, and/or referral.

- Participates in the development of written discharge instructions.

- Assists the patient and significant others in the identification of factors that place them "at risk" for illness or injury.

- Explains methods for illness or injury prevention, as appropriate.

Excellent Level

- Initiates development of alternative instructional methods, based on research.

- Evaluates and revises patient educational materials to accommodate diverse patient populations.

4. *The emergency nurse functions as a facilitator and liaison among health care providers and health care agencies, respecting their limits, abilities, and responsibilities.*

Competent Level

- Participates in multidisciplinary patient care conferences.

- Collaborates with other health care providers to make decisions for each patient's care.

- Identifies appropriate referral agencies to help meet patients' needs.

Excellent Level

- Participates in professional and community committees related to emergency care issues.

- Communicates with other specialty nursing organizations and other disciplines to address relevant issues.

- Demonstrates expertise in conflict resolution between patient and staff, staff and health care provider, and/or staff and staff.

Comprehensive Standard XIV
Research

ANA Standard*
The nurse uses research findings in practice.

Specialty Standard
The emergency nurse recognizes, supports, and utilizes research to enhance emergency nursing practice.

Rationale
Research is necessary to develop a body of validated nursing knowledge on which emergency nursing practice is based.

AMERICAN NURSES ASSOCIATION MEASUREMENT CRITERIA*

1. The nurse utilizes best available evidence, preferably research data, to develop the plan of care and interventions.

2. The nurse participates in research activities as appropriate to the nurse's education and position. Such activities may include:
   - identifying clinical problems suitable for nursing research
   - participating in data collection
   - participating in a unit, organization, or community research committee or program
   - sharing research activities with others
   - conducting research
   - critiquing research for application to practice
   - using research findings in the development of policies, procedures, and practice guidelines for patient care

* Reprinted with permission from American Nurses Association, *Standards of Clinical Nursing Practice*, *2nd edition.* ©1998 American Nurses Publishing, American Nurses Foundation/American Nurses Association, 600 Maryland Avenue, SW, Suite 100 West, Washington, DC 20024-2571.

EMERGENCY NURSES ASSOCIATION MEASUREMENT CRITERIA

1. The emergency nurse uses information from research literature to improve practice.

Competent Level

- Possesses current knowledge of current research in emergency care.

- Acts as an advocate for patients in the application of research findings to clinical practice.

- Critiques emergency care research.

- Shares research findings with peers.

Excellent Level

- Disseminates research findings to peers and colleagues through formal channels.

- Monitors literature for research pertaining to potential changes in nursing practice or the health care system.

- Develops and implements changes in practice in response to research.

- Develops and implements changes in the health care system in response to research.

2. The emergency nurse participates in research to expand the body of validated knowledge related to emergency nursing.

Competent Level

- Collects and records research data for approved studies in emergency nursing and care.

- Identifies clinical problems or questions for research related to emergency nursing and care.

- Acts as a patient advocate during the collection of research data.

Excellent Level

- Designs and implements collaborative research projects related to emergency nursing and care.

- Acts as a patient advocate by serving on review committees for the protection of human rights.

- Assists peers in identifying clinical problems for research in emergency nursing and care.

- Assists peers in designing and implementing research projects in emergency nursing and care.

- Incorporates findings of emergency nursing and care research into standards of practice for the setting.

- Pursues avenues for funding research.

- Initiates grant proposals for research projects in emergency care.

- Submits articles for publication regarding research findings.

3. The emergency nurse collaborates with colleagues in other disciplines engaged in research in the practice setting.

Competent Level

- Participates in and supports interdisciplinary research.
- Assists in identification of research subjects.

Excellent Level

- Initiates and facilitates interdisciplinary research.
- Maintains an awareness of current health care trends and shares this information with other health care providers.
- Communicates with legislators and/or regulatory agencies regarding health care issues, such as communicable diseases, trauma, or other specialized patient populations.
- Participates in the development of nursing interventions that minimize risk factors for illness or injury.

Comprehensive Standard XV
Resource Utilization

ANA Standard*
The nurse considers factors related to safety, effectiveness, and cost in planning and delivering patient care.

Specialty Standard
The emergency nurse collaborates with other health care providers to deliver patient- centered care in a manner consistent with safe, efficient, and cost-effective resource utilization.

Rationale
Emergency nurses have the professional responsibility to provide a safe environment and promote appropriate access to care in an efficient, cost-effective manner.

AMERICAN NURSES ASSOCIATION MEASUREMENT CRITERIA*

1. The nurse evaluates factors related to safety, effectiveness, availability, and cost when choosing between two or more practice options that would result in the same expected patient outcome.

2. The nurse assists the patient and family in identifying and securing appropriate and available services to address health-related needs.

3. The nurse assigns or delegates tasks as defined by the state nurse practice acts and according to the knowledge and skills of the designated caregiver.

4. If the nurse assigns or delegates tasks, it is based on the needs and condition of the patient, the potential for harm, the stability of the patient's condition, the complexity of the task, and the predictability of the outcome.

5. The nurse assists the patient and family in becoming informed consumers about the cost, risks, and benefits of treatment and care.

* Reprinted with permission from American Nurses Association, *Standards of Clinical Nursing Practice, 2nd edition.* ©1998 American Nurses Publishing, American Nurses Foundation/American Nurses Association, 600 Maryland Avenue, SW, Suite 100 West, Washington, DC 20024-2571.

EMERGENCY NURSES ASSOCIATION MEASUREMENT CRITERIA

1. The emergency nurse ensures that necessary supplies and equipment are readily available and appropriate charges are generated for their use.

Competent Level

- Ensures that supplies and equipment are readily available and in working order.
- Ensures delivery of efficient and effective care through assessment and evaluation of emergency facility operations.
- Documents emergency nursing activities in a way that supports the charges incurred by the patient.
- Ensures that charges to the patient are accurate and reflect the care that the patient received.
- Participates in appropriate product evaluation activities.

Excellent Level

- Recommends selection and utilization of supplies and equipment.
- Participates on product evaluation committees.
- Coordinates the maintenance and revision of patient charging systems within the department.

2. The emergency nurse takes appropriate measures to optimize the safety of peers, patients, significant others, other health care providers, and self in the emergency care setting.

Competent Level

- Demonstrates knowledge of standardized safety procedures in the emergency care setting.

- Identifies and rectifies sources of potential accidents through daily or periodic inspection.

- Implements safety procedures for each patient in accordance with that patient's specific needs.

- Demonstrates knowledge and compliance with practices that protect the healthcare provider and reduce the spread of infection in the emergency care setting.

- Demonstrates knowledge and skills necessary to implement the protocol to be followed in the event of an internal or external disaster or threat.

- Recognizes the potential for violence in the emergency setting and institutes appropriate action.

Excellent Level

- Participates in development of policies and procedures related to safety and bloodborne pathogens and Occupational Safety and Health Administration (OSHA) requirements.

- Coordinates education programs related to safety and bloodborne pathogens and OSHA requirements.

- Addresses violence in the emergency setting through the development, implementation, and evaluation of appropriate policies and procedures.

- Educates peers and other health care providers on management of violent situations.

- Participates in community education to increase awareness of violence as a health issue.

- Participates in the development of technology and utilization of products to enhance patient care and safety.

3. Assigns and delegates care that reflects the needs of patients and is in the scope of practice of other health care providers.

Competent Level

- Assigns and delegates care that reflects the needs of patients in the department.
- Alerts supervisory personnel to unsafe staffing situations.

Excellent Level

- Adjusts staffing requirements as changes occur in patient volumes, acuity, arrival times, and length of stay.

Glossary

Advanced Cardiac Life Support (ACLS®) A standardized course and verification process, under the auspices of the American Heart Association, that teaches interventions for identification and treatment of the patient in a cardio-pulmonary crisis. Includes airway management, dysrhythmia recognition and treatment, defibrillation, and pharmacology.

Assessment A systematic, dynamic process by which the nurse, through interaction with the client, significant others, and health care providers, collects and analyzes data about the client. Data may include the following dimensions: physical, psychosocial, spiritual, cognitive, functional abilities, developmental, economic, and lifestyle (ANA, 1998).

Basic Life Support (BLS®) A standardized course and verification process, under the auspices of the American Heart Association and the American Red Cross, that teaches interventions to support breathing and circulation for the patient who is pulseless and breathless. Includes chest compressions and rescue breathing.

Certification The process by which a professional is recognized for attainment and application of a specified body of emergency nursing knowledge.

Certified Emergency Nurse (CEN®) A registered professional nurse who has successfully passed the certification examination for emergency nurses. This examination measures attainment and application of a defined body of emergency nursing knowledge needed to function at a competent level.

Collaborative problem An actual or potential health problem that focuses on the pathophysiological response of the body and that nurses are responsible and accountable for identifying and treating in collaboration with the physician (Carpenito, 1992).

Competency based evaluation The system developed by an institution to assess each staff member's ability to meet performance expectations as stated in his or her job description.

Competent level The level of performance the emergency nurse or an institution should consider in establishing goals for the nurse's professional practice. Each area set forth in the standards does not necessarily have to be met for the nurse's performance to be competent. Competent emergency nursing is demonstrated by sound clinical judgment in autonomous practice.

Consolidated Omnibus Budget Reconciliation act of 1986 (COBRA) Legislation established to prevent patient dumping because of the lack of monetary resources.

Continuity of care An interdisciplinary process that includes clients and significant others in the development of a coordinated plan of care. The process facilitates the client's transition between settings, based on changing needs and available resources (ANA, 1998).

Course in Advanced Trauma Nursing: A Conceptual Approach (CATN) A 13-hour course developed to reinforce the interlocking psychophysiologic concepts central to trauma nursing. This course utilizes a case study approach to strengthen critical decision-making skills to optimally impact the outcome of critically injured patients.

Criteria Relevant, measurable indicators of the standards of clinical nursing practice (ANA, 1998).

Diagnosis A clinical judgment about the client's response to actual or potential health conditions or needs. Diagnoses provide basis for determination of a plan of care to achieve expected outcomes (ANA, 1998).

Diversity The ways in which people differ.

Emergency Medical Treatment and Active Labor Act (EMTALA) Federal legislation, formerly known as *COBRA*, passed by Congress to prevent patient dumping or transfer of unstable patients because of the lack of monetary resources.

Emergency Nurse Pediatric Course (ENPC) A 16-hour course, conducted under the auspices of the ENA, designed to provide core-level knowledge and psychomotor skills associated with the delivery of professional nursing care to the pediatric patient. This program has an optional verification component.

Emergency nursing The nursing assessment, diagnosis, and treatment of human responses to actual or potential, sudden or urgent, physical or psychosocial problems that are primarily episodic and acute in nature.

Entry level into practice The level of competence necessary for a nurse to begin practicing. It includes a registered nurse who is competent in basic nursing assessment and interventions but who continues to develop skills and expertise and develops knowledge-based judgments through experience and education.

Evaluation The process of determining both the patient's progress toward the attainment of expected outcomes and the effectiveness of nursing care (ANA, 1998).

Excellent level Practice that surpasses the competent level and contributes to the growth of emergency nursing practice.

Guidelines Describe a process of client care management which has the potential for improving the quality of clinical and consumer decision-making. Guidelines are systematically developed statements based on available scientific evidence and expert opinion (ANA, 1998).

Health care provider An individual with special expertise who provides health care services or assistance to clients. Providers may include nurses, physicians, paramedics, first responders, psychologists, social workers, nutritionists and dieticians, and various therapists. Providers also may include service organizations and vendors.

Implementation May include any or all of these activities: intervening, delegating, and coordinating. The client, significant others, or health care providers may be designated to implement interventions within the plan of care (ANA,1998).

Indicator A quantitative measure that can be used to collect and organize data about performance functions and processes related to patient care as well as care outcomes.

Medical screening examination The examination that the hospital would perform on any individual coming to the hospital emergency department with the same signs and symptoms within the capability of the hospital's emergency department, including ancillary services routinely available to the emergency department, to determine whether or not an emergency condition exists.

Nursing The diagnosis and treatment of human responses to actual or potential health problems (ANA, 1998).

Nursing diagnosis A clinical judgment about an individual, family, or community response to actual or potential health problems or life processes. Nursing diagnoses provide the basis for selection of nursing interventions to achieve outcomes for which the nurse is accountable (Carpenito, 1992).

Nursing Interventions Classification (NIC) The ordering or arranging of nursing activities into groups or sets on the basis of their relationships and assigning of intervention labels for the purpose of standardizing the language of nursing activities (McCloskey & Bulechek, 1992).

Nursing Outcomes Classification (NOC) The ordering or arranging of measurable, expected, client focused goals, as identified by the nurse, for the purpose of standardizing the language of nursing goals (Johnson & Maas, 1997).

Occupational Safety and Health Administration (OSHA) A federal regulatory agency established to promote safety in the workplace through mandated guidelines.

Outcome identification Measurable, expected, client-focused goals, as identified by the nurse through collaboration with the client and health care providers, when possible (ANA, 1998).

Patient Recipient of nursing actions. When the patient is an individual, the focus is on the health state, problems, or needs of a single person. When the patient is a family or group, the focus is on the health state of the unit as a whole or the reciprocal effects of an individual's health state on the other members of the unit. When the patient is a community, the focus is on personal and environmental health and the health risks of population groups. Nursing actions toward patients may be directed to disease or injury prevention, health promotion, health restoration, or health maintenance (ANA, 1998).

Pediatric Advanced Life Support (PALS®) Standardized 12-hour course and verification procedure, under the auspices of the American Heart Association and the American Academy of Pediatrics, to provide knowledge and skills for identification and management for cardio-pulmonary emergencies in the neonate and pediatric patient. Includes airway management, dysrhythmia recognition and treatment, defibrillation, venous access, and pharmacology.

Plan of care Comprehensive outline of care to be delivered to attain expected outcomes (ANA, 1998).

Rationale A justification for the standard.

Significant other A family member, parent, caregiver, and/or anyone who is significant to the patient.

Specialty Standard A standard that applies to all nurses practicing within a specific speciality setting. Specialty standards in this document apply to emergency nursing.

Standard Authoritative statement enunciated and promulgated by the profession and by which the quality of practice, service, or education can be judged (ANA, 1998).

Standards of Care Authoritative statements that describe a competent level of clinical nursing practice demonstrated through assessment, diagnosis, outcome identification, planning, implementation, and evaluation (ANA, 1998).

Standards of Professional Performance Authoritative statements that describe a competent level of behavior in the professional role, including activities related to quality of care, performance appraisal, education, collegiality, ethics, collaboration, research, and resource utilization (ANA, 1998).

Trauma Nursing Core Course (TNCC) A 16- or 20-hour course, conducted under the auspices of the ENA, designed to provide core-level trauma knowledge and psychomotor skills associated with the delivery of professional nursing care to the trauma patient. This program has an optional verification component.

Triage The process by which patients are evaluated and classified according to the type and urgency of their condition, for the purpose of determining treatment priorities. Patients are identified promptly using rapid assessments and interventions, to maintain the patient flow through the emergency department and provide information and referrals and to allay the anxieties of patients and significant others.

Wellness The optimum state of health and well being achieved through the utilization of measures to maintain health and prevent illness and/or injury.

Resources

American Heart Association. (1997). *Advanced cardiac life support*. Dallas: Author.

American Heart Association. (1997). *Basic life support for health care providers*. Dallas: Author.

American Heart Association. (1997). *Pediatric advanced life support*. Dallas: Author.

American Hospital Association. (1992). *A patient's bill of rights* (cat. No. 157759). Chicago: Author.

American Medical Association. (1992). Guidelines for cardiopulmonary resuscitation and emergency cardiac care. *Journal of the American Medical Association, 268* (16) 2171.

American Nurses Association. (1985). *Code for nurses with interpretive statements*. Washington, DC: Author.

American Nurses Association. (1995). *Nursing's social policy statement*. Washington, DC: Author.

American Nurses Association. (1998). *Standards of clinical nursing practice*. Washington, DC: Author.

Bloodborne Pathogens, 29 CFR § 1910.1030, (1995).

Carpenito, L. J. (1992). *Nursing diagnosis—application to clinical practice* (4th ed.). Philadelphia: J. B. Lippincott.

Consolidated Omnibus Budget Reconciliation Act (COBRA) of 1986, 42 USC § 1395dd, as amended by the Omnibus Budget Reconciliation Act (COBRA) of 1987, 1989, 1990, and 1994.

Emergency Medical Treatment and Active Labor Act, (EMTALA) 42 USC § 1395dd, (Suppl. 1995).

Emergency Nurses Association. (1992). *Emergency nurses guide to nursing diagnosis*. Park Ridge, IL: Author.

Emergency Nurses Association. (1993). *Orientation to emergency nursing: Diversity in practice.* Park Ridge, IL: Author.

Emergency Nurses Association. (1993). *Research initiatives.* Park Ridge, IL: Author.

Emergency Nurses Association. (1994). *Emergency nursing core curriculum* (4th ed.). Philadelphia: W. B. Saunders.

Emergency Nurses Association. (1995). *Course in advanced trauma nursing: A conceptual approach.* Park Ridge, IL: Author.

Emergency Nurses Association. (1995). *Emergency department patient classification manual* (2nd ed.). Park Ridge, IL: Author.

Emergency Nurses Association. (1995). *Trauma nursing core course* (3rd ed.). Park Ridge, IL: Author.

Emergency Nurses Association. (1996). *Advanced nursing practice manual.* Park Ridge, IL: Author.

Emergency Nurses Association. (1996). *About your emergency care.* Park Ridge, IL: Author.

Emergency Nurses Association. (1996). *Code of ethics for emergency nurses with interpretive statements.* Park Ridge, IL: Author.

Emergency Nurses Association. (1996). Position statement: Injury prevention. *ENA position statements* (pp. 61-70). Park Ridge, IL: Author.

Emergency Nurses Association. (1997). *Pediatric emergency nursing resource guide* (2nd ed.). Park Ridge, IL: Author.

Emergency Nurses Association. (1997). Position statement: Approaching diversity in emergency care. *ENA position statements* (pp. 11-12). Park Ridge, IL: Author.

Emergency Nurses Association. (1997). Position statement: Autonomous emergency nursing practice. *ENA position statements* (pp. 13-15). Park Ridge, IL: Author.

Emergency Nurses Association. (1997). Position statement: Bloodborne infectious diseases. *ENA position statements* (pp. 17-21). Park Ridge, IL: Author.

Emergency Nurses Association. (1997). Position statement: Chemical impairment of emergency nurses. *ENA position statements* (pp. 29-30). Park Ridge, IL: Author.

Emergency Nurses Association. (1997). Position statement: Collaborative and interdisciplinary research. *ENA position statements* (pp. 31-32). Park Ridge, IL: Author.

Emergency Nurses Association. (1997). Position statement: Enhanced 911 systems. *ENA position statements* (pp. 47-48). Park Ridge, IL: Author.

Emergency Nurses Association. (1997). Position statement: Hospital and emergency department overcrowding. *ENA position statements* (pp. 57-59). Park Ridge, IL: Author.

Emergency Nurses Association. (1997). Position statement: Interfacility transport of the critically ill or injured patient. *ENA position statements* (pp. 73-74). Park Ridge, IL: Author.

Emergency Nurses Association. (1997). Position statement: Observation/holding areas. *ENA position statements* (pp. 85-86). Park Ridge, IL: Author.

Emergency Nurses Association. (1997). Position statement: Protection of animal subjects. *ENA position statements* (pp. 91-92). Park Ridge, IL: Author.

Emergency Nurses Association. (1997). Position statement: Protection of human subjects' rights. *ENA position statements* (pp. 93-94). Park Ridge, IL: Author.

Emergency Nurses Association. (1997). Position statement: Staffing and productivity in the emergency care setting. *ENA position statements* (pp. 115-118). Park Ridge, IL: Author.

Emergency Nurses Association. (1997). Position statement: The use of non-registered nurse (non-RN) caregivers in emergency care. *ENA position statements* (pp. 133-138). Park Ridge, IL: Author.

Emergency Nurses Association. (1997). Position statement: Treatment of sexual assault survivors. *ENA position statements* (pp. 139-141). Park Ridge, IL: Author.

Emergency Nurses Association. (1997). Position statement: Violence in the emergency care setting. *ENA position statements* (pp. 147-151). Park Ridge, IL: Author.

Emergency Nurses Association. (1997). *Legislative manual* (3rd ed.). Park Ridge, IL: Author.

Emergency Nurses Association. (1997). *Triage: Meeting the challenge* (2nd ed.). Park Ridge, IL: Author.

Emergency Nurses Association. (1998). Position statement: Access to care. *ENA position statements* (pp. 3-5). Park Ridge, IL: Author.

Emergency Nurses Association. (1998). Position statement: Advanced practice in emergency nursing. *ENA position statements* (pp. 7-9). Park Ridge, IL: Author.

Emergency Nurses Association. (1998). Position statement: CEN® review courses and resource material. *ENA position statements* (pp. 27-28). Park Ridge, IL: Author.

Emergency Nurses Association. (1998). Position statement: Conscious sedation. *ENA position statements* (pp. 33-34). Park Ridge, IL: Author.

Emergency Nurses Association. (1998). Position statement: Critical incident stress management. *ENA position statements* (pp. 35-36). Park Ridge, IL: Author.

Emergency Nurses Association. (1998). Position statement: Domestic violence. *ENA position statements* (pp. 39-43). Park Ridge, IL: Author.

Emergency Nurses Association. (1998). Position statement: Integration of emergency nursing concepts in nursing curricula. *ENA position statements* (pp. 71-72). Park Ridge, IL: Author.

Emergency Nurses Association. (1998). Position statement: Resuscitative decisions. *ENA position statements* (pp. 95-96). Park Ridge, IL: Author.

Emergency Nurses Association. (1998). Position statement: Role of the emergency nurse in tissue and organ donation. *ENA position statements* (pp. 103-105). Park Ridge, IL: Author.

Emergency Nurses Association. (1998). Position statement: Role of the registered nurse in the prehospital environment. *ENA position statements* (pp. 107-111). Park Ridge, IL: Author.

Emergency Nurses Association. (1998). Position statement: Substance abuse. *ENA position statements* (pp. 119-120). Park Ridge, IL: Author.

Emergency Nurses Association. (1998). Position statement: Telephone advice. *ENA position statements* (pp. 121-123). Park Ridge, IL: Author.

Emergency Nurses Association. (1998). [Graduate programs offering emergency- or trauma-related nursing tracks]. Unpublished raw data.

Emergency Nurses Association. (1999). *Emergency nursing pediatric course.* Park Ridge, IL: Author.

Johnson, M., & Maas, M., (Eds.). (1997). Iowa Outcomes Project. *Nursing outcomes classification* (NOC). St. Louis: Mosby.

McCloskey, J. C., & Bulechek, G. M., (Eds.) (1992). Iowa Intervention Project. *Nursing interventions classification (NIC).* St. Louis: Mosby.

Joint Commission on Accreditation of Healthcare Organizations. (1998). *Comprehensive accreditation manual for hospitals: The official handbook.* Oakbrook Terrace, IL: Author.